HOW TO ROCK YOUR SMILE

A Patient's Guide to Perfect Health through a Perfect Smile!

By Dr. Boyd O. Whitlock III

Mission Statement

At WHITLOCK ORTHODONTICS,
our mission is to **efficiently** create long lasting smiles.

We are committed to providing the highest level of
care by utilizing educational and technological **growth** in
a **fun, positive atmosphere.**

We strive to encompass superior **integrity** and genuine
character within our team. As a family, we are
committed to giving back and leaving a strong
community legacy.

Rock Your Smile

W
Whitlock
Orthodontics

THANK YOU

I want to say thank you to the following people who inspired and supported me in writing this book:

First of all, my family has inspired me and supported me most of all. At the time of this book's publication, this has involved

    Karen Whitlock
    Alyssa Whitlock
    Kylie Whitlock
    Bo Whitlock

Eddie Coleman (friend and mentor)

Dr. Lun Wang (colleague and fellow best-seller)

Ramy Habeeb (writing coach)

My Purpose

Growing up, I had braces four different times, along with two jaw surgeries. Because of trauma to my mouth, I have also had almost every dental procedure possible—and I would do it all again. I understand the value of a great smile. It has given me great confidence to enter the world. I have found it so life-changing that I want to help others achieve the same.

To accomplish this, after four years of college, then four years of dental school, I completed a three-year orthodontic residency.

I decided to write this book to help you understand everything involved in getting a great smile, a perfect smile, a healthy smile—to Rock Your Smile. I have included topics, terms, and procedures that I believe to be necessary and helpful, using a doctor's knowledge base and explaining it from a patient's perspective.

I hope you enjoy it and find it helpful!

TABLE OF CONTENTS

TRACK 1:

MY STORY—WHY I'M WRITING A BOOK

Have you ever sat in a movie theater, looked up at the screen, and seen that movie star with that gorgeous white smile? You thought to yourself, "Wow! She has a really pretty smile ... I wish mine looked like that!"

Or perhaps you've been sitting at dinner with some friends, and thought to yourself, "Oh my goodness ... I wish I had a smile like they have!"

You're not alone.

Hopefully, by the time you finish this book, you'll understand what is involved to help you take your ordinary smile and improve it so you can Rock Your Smile!

You may be wondering why I wrote this book. Let me start by telling you a little of my story.

I grew up in the Midwest in a medical family—my dad was a physician and my mom was a nurse—so we had a lot of "doctor talk" around the dinner table.

Growing up, my uncle was my orthodontist. I loved the impact that a pretty smile had in my life. I wanted to do that for others! So I decided at a young age that I wanted to be an orthodontist. My younger brother eventually became a plastic surgeon, and my little sister followed in our mother's footsteps and became a nurse. We definitely grew up in a healthcare environment.

I'm writing this book from both a doctor's perspective as well as from a patient's perspective. Because my uncle was my orthodontist, I ended up with braces early on—I think I was around ten years old. Back in that time, in the early '70s (I know, for a lot you that's a long time ago), the majority of the kids did not get braces. At that time, there was not yet a big emphasis on facial esthetics. So because there was not a real perceived value in most cases, they were too expensive for the average person. Plus, they were big, metal, and bulky—not very socially "cool." But because my uncle was an orthodontist, I was one of the "lucky ones" that got braces (I didn't consider it lucky at the time).

I got my braces off after a couple of years. But, unfortunately, my lower jaw kept growing, and I again had an underbite. In eighth grade, I ended up with braces again (perfect timing back then for a boy who was already going through puberty to also add "train tracks" and glasses). This time I had to have four teeth taken out to try to correct my underbite. So after another two-plus years, I got them off right after I got my driver's license (great—big "Metal Mouth" on my license for the next four years!). They attributed this continued growth pattern to my genetics (both my grandma and my dad had a big chin), and in second grade I broke my nose, which probably affected the growth of my upper jaw.

My junior year was an awesome year—no braces! Although, I did have that old-fashioned retainer with the wire around your teeth that made you talk with a lisp ... But still—no big metal braces!

But then, during my senior year, my underbite started showing back up again. That year they had just started doing jaw surgeries, which I'd really needed from the beginning. At that time, they were only doing lower jaw surgery. So guess who got braces for a *third* time? Yes, a third time? That's right—yours truly. My lower jaw was still growing (why couldn't my height have continued to grow as well?). I got braces on at the end of my senior year (yes—before graduation) and started college with braces. I had my lower jaw moved back some over Christmas break of my freshman year. I finally got them off that summer, allowing me to start my sophomore year of college without braces.

You won't believe what happened next. One night, I was helping set up for the opening of a local waterpark and we were moving picnic tables, in the dark. The guy carrying the front of the table stepped into a hole and dropped the table. The next thing I knew, I was flat on my back, surrounded by all of my co-workers. I felt with my tongue and discovered that I had fractured off my front teeth. I ended up with root canals, crowns, and eventually an implant.

Several years later, while I was in my orthodontic residency, I realized I needed surgery on my upper jaw as well. But I was in school, didn't have time or money, yada, yada, yada. Finally, after I had been in practice for several years, I decided I had to put my money where my mouth was (for *real* in this case). I went back into braces for the fourth time—yes, the *fourth* time—and had my second jaw surgery.

To this day, I still hold the record in my practice, and I'm proud to keep that record—four times in braces!

For those of you that paid attention, you probably realized that, yes, I had braces in elementary school, junior high, high school *and* college; and every important life event for a kid—junior high, driver's license, prom, high school graduation. I could have played a great character in a TV show.

So let's review my history: braces four times, two jaw surgeries, a filling, a crown, a root canal, tooth extraction, gum graft, bone graft, implant, and a septoplasty to fix my broken nose. Now take a moment to flip back to the "About the Author" page. Check out that smile! Needless to say, I know what it takes to get a Rock Star Smile from a patient's perspective. After four years of college (BS in Psychology), four years of dental school (DDS—Doctorate in Dental Surgery), a one-year General Practice Residency (GPR), then three years of Orthodontic Residency (Orthodontic Certificate and MSOB), I have the education background to figure out what it takes to help you Rock Your Smile. About everything there is you could possibly need to do to get your Rock Star Smile, I've had done. My undergraduate degree was Psychology; therefore, I also understand and appreciate the psychological aspect, besides just the functional, of how important it is for someone to feel good about themselves. Like I said, my brother is a plastic surgeon, and my sister is a nurse and runs a med-spa. Aesthetics and feeling good about yourself are important to our whole family.

I approach every patient as if they are my own family member. It is important to me to make an impact on everyone that God brings across my path, to improve his or her total physical and psychological health. That's what this book is about—how to achieve total health, both physical and psychological, and being able to smile, not only with straight, pretty teeth, but also from the inside out.

Now ... Let's Rock Your Smile!

TRACK 2:

WHAT MAKES UP A ROCK STAR SMILE

So you want to Rock Your Smile.

You want to have that Rock Star Smile, that Hollywood smile, a smile you can be proud of. A smile that will give you the confidence to achieve whatever you want out of life. A smile that might help you even get married ... (*wink, wink*). A smile that will last a lifetime.

So what makes up a Rock Star Smile? What defines a pretty smile? Years ago, many artists such as Leonardo Da Vinci defined a pretty face as being balanced, following studied proportions, defined aesthetic qualities, following defined curves. I'll go through some of these in common folks' terms. I'll explain how these definitions are used to find that balance and get your Rock Star Smile.

First of all, we have to talk about the foundation. The foundation of a gorgeous Rock Star Smile is having balanced proportions between the left and right sides of your face. We know that none of us are perfectly symmetrical. You've probably seen pictures—or even did this yourself—of someone holding up a mirror in the middle of their face. The mirrored image of their right side and the mirrored image of their left side look like two different people. Nevertheless, to have a Rock Star Smile, the two sides have to be close, balanced, and proportioned.

Second, even though we don't see our own profile except in picture, we have to make sure that we are balanced in a proper proportion from the upper and lower jaw, not only front to back, but also in height. Do we have too big of a chin? Too short an upper lip? Those are important, and should be evaluated. Those are the foundational structures.

Next, we start looking at the surface. We look at the eyes. Are they balanced, level, and equal? Are we getting good rest? Then we evaluate the nose. Is it straight, tipped up, or down? Is it narrow or broad? We are interested in whether or not someone appears to be resting well and breathing properly.

We then look at the lips. Is there symmetry? Is there a scar? Is there good fullness to them? Can we get them closed together over the teeth? How do the lips move when we smile? Do they move too far, showing too much gum tissue? Do they move up more on one side, giving an unsymmetrical appearance?

Finally, we move to the teeth. First, how do they fit in our face? How broad of a smile do we have and how do our teeth fit within our smile—too narrow, too full, or just right? When we smile, is it guarded? Meaning, are we restraining from a "full" smile because we haven't been happy with our teeth in the past? Then, we look at the position of the teeth. Are the teeth straight? Are the teeth themselves pretty in color and shape? What about the width of the upper jaw? Does it fill out the width of our smile? Do our upper teeth follow our lower lip (a good "smile arc").

We'll go into each of these sections as we go throughout this book, but those are many of the aspects of what make up an aesthetic smile.

TRACK 3:

WHAT IS ORTHODONTICS?

You might be asking, "What is orthodontics? What does an orthodontist do?"

Orthodontics used to be called *orthodontia*—the word comes from the Greek words *orthos*, meaning "straight, perfect, or proper," and *dontos*, which means "teeth."

Orthodontics is a branch of dentistry that specializes in treating patients with improper positioning of teeth when the mouth is closed (malocclusion), which results in an improper bite. It is a dental specialty degree, requiring two to three years of further education after graduating from dental school. An orthodontics specialist is called an orthodontist.

The field of orthodontics also includes treating and controlling various aspects of facial growth (dentofacial orthopedics) and the shape and development of the jaw. Orthodontics also includes cosmetic dentistry, when the patient's aim is to improve his/her appearance.

Dentofacial orthopedics is the process of normalizing the growth of a patient's bone structure and repairing any imbalances of the face and jaws. This process often involves a two-phase treatment and often begins before the patient is seven years old.

As I shared with you earlier, I had braces four times. I grew up thinking that I wanted to be an orthodontist. It had such an impact on me by giving me a pretty smile and giving me my self-confidence that I wanted to be able to help others get pretty smiles and get that self-confidence.

So I started on this journey to be an orthodontist thinking that it was all about creating pretty, straight teeth. The idea of taking someone that wouldn't smile because of his or her crooked, ugly teeth and be able to give them a pretty smile seemed very rewarding to me—and life-changing to anyone that I could help.

Well, as I have learned throughout my years as an orthodontist, it takes *so* much more than just straight teeth to create a pretty smile. Now, don't get me wrong—straight teeth are certainly prettier than crooked, but they aren't the best. Straight teeth are not the only thing needed to create a pretty smile, a Rock Star Smile, to allow you to Rock Your Smile.

You also need a balanced and proportioned face. This is where the proper and thorough evaluation of your skeletal structure comes in. This process has drastically improved now with our ability to evaluate your jaws and facial structures using our digital 3D imaging.

With my family background and my commitment to healthcare, I have built my practice as more than just a "tooth straightener." I am also a healthcare provider, and I am dedicated in doing whatever I can to improve a person's total health.

Types of Orthodontic Therapy:

Many of you as old as me might remember the old metal bands that had to go all the way around each tooth. Remember being called "Metal Mouth" or "Train Tracks"? Well, great news for anyone needing orthodontic therapy today (especially at Whitlock Orthodontics)! Remember, I had braces four times—so my passion today to create a better experience for you means shorter treatment times, less discomfort, and better overall facial results.

New Brackets:

Now we have much smaller and smoother brackets that are bonded or attached to your tooth structure. We use brackets that have a "little door" that helps hold in the wires. This provides more comfort—lighter force, and no pokey wires—and better oral hygiene.

We have esthetic options: clear brackets and "lingual brackets." Lingual brackets are braces that we can now bond on the inside of your teeth make it so no one sees them at all. Because of our computerized planning, where we use special CAD/CAM computer software to plan out your smile, lingual braces have finally become a real possibility.

We also offer clear aligner therapy (Invisalign). Aligner therapy is planned on a CAD/CAM computer software. The movement is staged step-by-step. A new aligner is then made at each stage. Therefore, with a series of aligners, your teeth can be moved to their planned alignment position one stage at a time. The advantage of aligners is that they are clear, so no one knows you have them in. Because you can take them in and out, you can take them out to eat—which means you can eat whatever you want!

NEW TECHNOLOGIES:

SURESMILE—Remember, one of my goals is to reduce the amount of time that you are in braces. There are many new technologies coming out every year. I have selected the best options with this goal in mind. In 2004, I was introduced to a computerized CAD/CAM software that allows me to position your teeth in the proper alignment and the position that would be the best fit for your smile, for your face. Then, once the positioning is satisfactory, this data is sent to a robot that custom bends our archwires, providing a customized, individualized archwire just for you.

We are one of the first in the country to adopt this incredible technology. As a result, we have become a world leader in 3D digital treatment. I have taught hundreds of other orthodontists around the world how to use this technology to improve the quality of care they provide to their patients.

Not only has SureSmile allowed us to provide better care, but it has followed our goals by allowing us to reduce our treatment times, the time you will be in braces. The national average is somewhere around 28 months (many of us remember ours as much longer than that). Using (and mastering) the SureSmile system has allowed us to reduce our treatment times down to about fourteen months—almost in half! We have also reduced the number of trips that require you to get out of school, or off work, by almost 40 percent.

As someone who spent most of my pre-teen, teenage and young adult life in braces, I find this very exciting!

MICRO-PULSES:

We have also found and incorporated a device that you can use that uses micro- pulses to temporarily change the bone morphology to assist in even more rapid tooth movement. This is reducing our treatment times by another 30 percent.

This combined with our SureSmile and 3D planning means we can get your braces on and off in less than twelve months ... *WOW!* That sounds awesome, huh?

As you can see, we have found many new advantages; I am further committed to continue to follow and try new technologies and treatment options to reduce your time in braces.

TRACK 4:

WHEN SHOULD I START?

You might be asking yourself, "When should I take my kid to see the orthodontist?"

Or you might be thinking, "But isn't he too young? I don't want to have to do it again ..."

These are excellent questions.

They are also both very popular common questions that we get. People ask each other, ask their friends, and a lot of times they're told, even by their general dentist, "Oh, just wait until all of the permanent (or 'grown-up') teeth come in." What we have seen, and what the research now shows, is that this is generally true. Waiting until all the permanent teeth come in will still allow for good tooth alignment. If that's all that you are interested in, then that is a good time to come in to simply straighten up all your teeth.

BUT ...

My core values, my beliefs, are to treat you and/or your child the same way I would treat my own family members. Which means I would have to say, "Don't wait!"

When I started looking at my kids as they were growing, I noticed a couple of things as they turned five and six years old.

First, their jaws weren't matching up and growing properly. Second, they were not breathing very well at night. They were struggling to concentrate at school, restless at nighttime, and I noticed they sometimes snored when I would check in on them. Because they were my kids and I had some concerns about their overall health, I began looking at them a little earlier than what had been recommended in the literature and by the "old guard" orthodontists at that time.

I started researching for answers to my questions, like "Why would a kid's growth pattern be off?" What I found was that for some, it can be their genetics. Perhaps their dad or mom or grandpa or uncle has a jaw growth problem, and it's inherited. My dad and other family members have a "strong chin," a potential toward an underbite. So I have a genetic potential.

There can also be an environmental cause. What happens around us as we grow up can have an impact on us. We know that allergies and mouth breathing can modify the growth; trauma, or some other occurrence, can also change the normal growth pattern for an individual. For me personally, that was one of the factors. When I was only seven years old, I was hit in the face with a ball that broke my nose. This, combined with when I fell and fractured my teeth, impacted the growth of my upper jaw. Add to this my genetic or family tendency toward an underbite, and I had a jaw growth discrepancy. Jaw growth is one thing that we look at during our initial visit, especially with young growing children.

First we look at jaw growth, and second we look at tooth development and eruption. Using the latest 3D imaging, we are now able to evaluate whether all of the teeth are present, how they are erupting (or growing), and if they are erupting in the proper place. During this initial, early stage of a kid's growth, we are also measuring if there is going to be enough room for all the teeth to come in. With this information, we decide if we need to do anything at this time, or if we should wait.

The third thing that's important to evaluate at this age, and probably one of the most important things for me, is the airway. Like I mentioned earlier, when my kids went to sleep, they were restless and tossing. This began to make me think about airway. Recently research has come out showing many kids diagnosed with ADD and ADHD may be showing symptoms related to sleep airway problems. We can observe and evaluate sinuses and nasal passages, and tonsils and adenoids, make referrals when necessary, and modify skeletal growth at an early age to assist in opening the airway.

Going back to modifying growth: we can increase the space for the tongue. I can help get the tongue out of the back of the throat, and therefore help them breathe better by expanding or widening the upper and lower teeth. We also help open the nasal air passages when we widen the upper jaw. Obviously, this is an important time in your kid's life. First, it is important that your kid is breathing and getting enough oxygen; but we also know that this is an important time in their cognitive development. This is not something that we can wait for, and it is something that we need to do as soon as possible.

The fourth thing that is important to do at an early age is to make sure there is proper space for all of the adult teeth to come in. At this early age, we can modify the growth in order to open space and create an easier situation for the teeth to have room to erupt. It makes our "braces time" shorter. I think we can all agree it would be best to reduce the length of Phase II, since this usually happens during their teenage years—and we all know teenagers are a little more difficult to get along with.

That's my goal. I truly believe that early treatment is important for increasing the airway and providing adequate jaw growth for proper tooth eruption.

Fifth is looking at cooperation. A lot of people, including a lot of orthodontists, will say, "Just wait. Let's do it all in the full braces phase, or when they get older. We can get the same results then." The first problem with this plan is, as I mentioned previously, when you consider the potential health risks, we can't afford to wait. My second problem with waiting is there are some facial changes that we can make at an earlier stage that just aren't possible in the later stage without either teeth removal or surgery.

At the very least, even if the patient is not ready for any treatment, we can start to educate and inform the parent as to what they can expect and when it might be.

With this in mind, our goals for early treatment, or Phase I, are the following:

1. Using our 3D imaging—we look at the child's airways. Is the child growing and developing as he/she should be? We look to see if the jaw bones are growing as they should be and if the teeth are growing and developing on schedule and with adequate space.
2. If they are not, is there something we need to do at this time?
3. If we decide we need to treat at this time, then we decide what type of treatment is needed to modify growth of the jaws and teeth. There are lots of different appliances and techniques that we can use to modify their growth pattern.

TRACK 5:

WHY AIRWAY?

Why am I talking about airway? Why is an *orthodontist* talking about airway? Why would I dedicate a whole chapter in this book to discuss obstructive airway issues? Well, as I've said, I am passionate about helping you Rock Your Smile, based on improving your total body health. If you are having problems breathing, during the day or especially at night, you are not at optimum health—which means you aren't able to Rock Your Smile as well!

Obstructive sleep apnea (OSA) and airway issues have touched me personally in several ways. As a kid I had difficulty in breathing—allergies, broken nose, deviated septum, etc. Of course, no one asked about or was aware of this (even me) until I had some procedures that improved my breathing; then and only then did I realize that I hadn't been breathing very well before.

Years later, I noticed that my children were restless at night and sometimes didn't sleep very well and had a difficult time paying attention, especially in school. After their orthodontic treatment, including expansion, their symptoms improved. Still, nobody was discussing this connection back then.

Recently, my mother passed away. She had weight management issues most of her life, which caused, among other things, heart issues and type 2 diabetes. She was diagnosed with OSA and was prescribed a CPAP machine to wear at night. Remember, she was an RN and my dad a physician, and yet she did not consistently wear her CPAP. Only near the end of her life, when helping her into bed and trying to hook up her CPAP for her, did I realize that when she did wear it, it was not being used properly. She didn't like how tight it fit on her face and the marks she would wake up with. Due to this, she wasn't breathing well; she had related health issues and she knew better.

So I am *very* passionate about making a difference in people's total health—not just straightening their teeth.

Obstructive Sleep Apnea

"What is obstructive sleep apnea, or OSA? And why should I care? How do I know if I have it?" These are all great and very common questions.

What Is Sleep Apnea?

When you have this condition, your breath can become very shallow; you may even stop breathing briefly while you sleep. It can happen many times a night in some cases.

Obstructive sleep apnea happens when something partly or completely blocks your upper airway during shut-eye. This makes your diaphragm and chest muscles work harder to open the obstructed airway and pull air into the lungs. Breathing usually resumes with a loud gasp, snort, or body jerk. You may not sleep well, but you probably won't be aware that this is happening.

This condition can also reduce the flow of oxygen to vital organs and cause irregular heart rhythms.

Symptoms

The most common obstructive sleep apnea warning signs include:

Adults

- Daytime sleepiness or fatigue
- Dry mouth or sore throat when you wake up
- Headaches in the morning
- Trouble concentrating, forgetfulness, depression, or irritability
- Night sweats

- Restlessness during sleep
- Problems with sex
- Snoring
- Waking up suddenly and feeling like you're gasping or choking
- Trouble getting up in the mornings

If you share a bed with someone, they'll probably notice it before you do.

Kids

Symptoms in children may not be as obvious. They may include:

- Bedwetting
- Choking or drooling
- Sweating a lot at night
- Ribcage moves inward when they exhale
- Learning and behavior disorders
- Problems at school
- Sluggishness or sleepiness (often misinterpreted as laziness in the classroom)
- Snoring
- Teeth grinding (bruxism)
- Restlessness in bed
- Pauses or absence of breathing
- Unusual sleeping positions, such as sleeping on the hands and knees, or with the neck hyperextended

Who Gets Obstructive Sleep Apnea?

According to a recent Harvard health report, approximately 25 million adults in the US suffer from OSA—and almost nineteen million of them are undiagnosed. OSA is more likely if you are overweight or have a thick or large neck, or have smaller airways in your nose, throat, or mouth. It can also happen if you have enlarged tonsils or too much tissue at the back of the throat—the uvula and soft palate—that hangs down and blocks the windpipe. A larger-than-average tongue can also block the airway in many people, as well as a deviated septum in the nose.

The condition is more common among men than women, and it becomes more likely as you get older. But it's not a normal part of aging.

Other risk factors include:

- Smoking
- Type 2 diabetes
- High blood pressure
- Being at risk for heart failure or stroke

Diagnosis

Although the final diagnosis must be made by a physician using a sleep study, we can now screen many patients, especially kids, and help prevent them from suffering from sleep breathing problems.

What are potential risks if left untreated?

1. Adults
   a. High blood pressure
   b. Coronary artery disease
   c. Stroke
   d. Congestive heart failure
   e. Heart attack
   f. Atrial fibrillation
   g. Restless leg syndrome
2. Children
   a. Diagnosed as ADD, ADHD
   b. Decreased cognitive development
   c. Active sleep

What are treatment options?

CPAP:

Still at the time of this writing, the primary recommendation for someone diagnosed with obstructive sleep is a CPAP. Most likely, you have heard of a CPAP but might not be entirely familiar with it. This device includes a mask that you must wear over your nose, mouth, or sometimes both. It has an air blower that forces constant and continuous air through your nose and/or mouth. The seal of the mask must be tight enough with sufficient pressure from the blower to force open your airway and inflate your lungs during sleep. Other types of positive airway pressure devices are also available, including the BPAP, which has two levels of air flow that vary with breathing in and out.

The advantage of using a CPAP is that it forces air into your lungs and gets you breathing. The disadvantages are that most people are too intimidated to even go get tested with a sleep study—they don't want to pay to have someone watch them sleep, and they don't want to be told they need a CPAP. The CPAP also has to be maintained, cleaned, and hoses replaced periodically. You also have to wear it, which is inconvenient when traveling, when napping on the coach, etc.

Oral Appliances:

The next therapy recommended, and growing in popularity, is an oral appliance. When a dentist/orthodontist has been properly trained, they can make an appliance that holds the lower jaw forward, and therefore the tongue forward, thereby opening the airway while sleeping.

The advantage of the sleep appliance is that there is no machine to keep up with, maintain, travel with, etc. They are easier to sleep with, travel with. The disadvantage is that they still have to be worn to be effective. If they are forgotten, if you fall asleep on the couch, etc., then you don't have it in. The appliance can move the teeth and therefore change the bite. This is why an orthodontist needs to be involved with delivering a sleep appliance. They know both how to reduce the amount of tooth movement and how to correct it if it does happen.

Surgical correction:

By combining orthodontics and jaw surgery, both the upper and lower jaws are widened and brought forward, resulting in an increased airway.

The advantage is that this is a physical, permanent change. You don't have to remember to keep up with a nighttime appliance. The disadvantage is that it is a surgical procedure. There are the usual potential risks when anyone has a surgery, and the cost of having both jaws operated on is sometimes outside someone's budget.

Adult Orthodontics:

Many times we can widen the teeth inside the upper and lower jaws. This gives your tongue more space to rest forward, resulting in an increased airway.

Kids' airway-centric orthodontic:

This is similar to what other orthodontists might use, but with the focus being on increasing the child's airway, improving their total body health. When we see that the airway is narrow, we evaluate their tonsils and adenoids and give referrals if we see that they might be a problem. Then we expand/widen the arches and help the lower jaw grow more. This both helps move the tongue forward and results in opening the airway. Our goal is to help the child breathe better to help them not lose some of their cognitive development. It is also to help keep them from developing OSA later in their life.

This is so important to me! Please make sure that you and your child have your airways evaluated and treated if needed. It's what we do—help you improve your total body health and get you to Rock Your Smile!

TRACK 6:

HEADACHES & MIGRAINES

It was a cool fall day in October in Tulsa, OK. I was eight years old and in third grade. I remember riding my cool banana-seat bicycle home from school.

Normally, my mom would welcome me home with a hug. On this particular day, I remember, she wasn't there at the door, but was laying on the couch, asleep. I was worried about her and kissed her on the cheek and told her I was home.

She said, "OK, baby. Please check on your little brother and sister, and you all please be quiet. I am trying to get rid of this bad headache."

Throughout my childhood years, I remember several occasions where my mom either suffered through particular events or stayed home and missed the event entirely due to a headache. As a young child, I didn't know what else to do but to leave her alone and hope her medicine helped her sleep it off.

Jump forward fifteen years. I am engaged to my fiancée, Karen. I was in dental school and she was finishing up her college degree. I remember coming home late from school and coming to her parents' house to find her laying downstairs in the dark. Her mom said she had a migraine and she had taken her prescription medicine. I went down to check on her and found her throwing up in the bathroom. This was a frequent occurrence for her because of the severe pain (possibly also a side effect of the medication).

As mentioned earlier, I grew up in the medical world. I had complete faith that the medical world was doing whatever it could with care and compassion to take care of and treat these two important ladies. In dental school, I studied the anatomy and physiology of the head and neck environment, and I began questioning that maybe the medical world didn't have all of the information to adequately solve the problem of suffering from severe headaches.

According to the World Health Organization, one out of every twenty people in the world suffers with daily headaches. Over 12 percent of North Americans suffer from migraines every year. Well over 100 million workdays are lost annually to headaches—and who knows how many personal events and activities have been missed. It appears that we have a "headache epidemic" on our hands. Even with all our advances in modern medicine, and the numerous kinds of treatments for headaches, there is still a large group of chronic head-pain patients who have eluded all conventional medical treatments.

Why have we not found a cure for headaches?

Most of us will initially seek out a physician when we have chronic headaches and migraines, which in most cases is the right place to start. We want to eliminate any potential severe medical condition that might be the cause. However, evidence shows that over 80 percent of pain conditions in the head and neck area actually involve the mouth and the jaw. A large percentage of these chronic headaches and migraines are related to injuries resulting from improper forces associated with the muscles, joints, and other soft tissues in the oral cavity and in the head and neck area.

Up until now, there has not been a good way to properly assess these patients and their pain. This is why some treatments will work for one patient and not for others. The breakthrough came when we realized that we must combine the expertise of advanced dentistry and medical rehabilitation techniques in order to address the needs of patients with this type of head pain. By combining new technology from both dentistry and medicine, we can now properly identify the area of injury and provide proper treatment for these patients. Dentists, with their basic medical background and thorough knowledge of the head and neck area, are the clear and obvious choice to perform these assessments and then deliver the proper treatment.

Many patients view the idea of a dentist treating their chronic headaches with skepticism and doubt. They desperately want to find relief, but have been disappointed and let down so many times before, that they guard themselves against getting their hopes up. So many have given up hope. They believe, as many in the medical world have told them, that they will just have to "live with it."

The single most common initiating cause for dentomandibular sensorimotor dysfunction (DMSD) patients' pain to become chronic and complex is motor vehicle accidents, followed by work-related injuries. Preexisting conditions from a list of common orofacial pain conditions may also exist to varying degrees, creating the patient's unique and complicated pain profile.

Treatment by experts in the medical field, however, rarely consider areas in and around the oral cavity. Therefore, many of the imbalances described in DMSD are not addressed, and their "buckets" are still full.

1. History
2. Must have medical back up
3. Inside and out
4. Muscle palpation
5. TMJ assessment
6. Dental assessment
7. Dental force analysis
8. Range of motion

A dentist and dental specialist (including an orthodontist) are often the best choice for assessment and treatment of head pain. Not only are we well versed in the anatomy and physiology of this area, we alone among the entire healthcare professionals are able to combine expertise in medicine, physical therapy, rehabilitative therapy, and advance dentistry for treatments in the head and neck area. This is not to say that we should be the only healthcare provider to treat all headaches. Far from it. There are causes to headaches that only a medical professional can diagnose and treat; however they are a relative small percentage by occurrence.

The typical patient that I have seen in my practice has chronic pain. They usually present me with one or more of the following:

1. They have had pain anywhere from as little as three months to more than 25 years
2. They have seen a family physician and usually other specialists
3. They have not had long-term success with any previously recommended treatment
4. Many have tried alternative medicine (natural, herbal, etc.)
5. Most have tried many different drugs. Either the drugs have not worked or have too many side effects to continue using

The design of our assessment protocol is to tease out all the areas of possible pain production. This thorough examination covers all the areas of head and neck and oral cavity. The results give us a list of probable causes of the head pain. As previously mentioned, the bucket analogy dictates that we need to find as many of the factors as possible to reduce or eliminate pain on a long-term basis. At the end of this examination, we are able to create a problem list that covers diseases and disorders that span the field of medicine and dentistry that can cause pain. With this list, a plan can be created that will address as many of the problems in the "bucket," to achieve effective and lasting results.

Since a large percentage of the complex chronic pain patients have their problems originate from traumatic events, the imbalances in their system are usually from undiagnosed and untreated injuries. I asked myself, Who on earth receives the best rehabilitative care? My answer? Professional athletes. Since they are paid millions of dollars to perform, it stands to reason that they get the most technologically advanced treatment for recovery. Have you heard of a football player who broke a leg or tore a shoulder only to recover and come back within weeks of the injury to perform at the height of their abilities again? Well, I can tell you that when I damaged my knee, it took me two months to see a knee specialist, and another three months to get an MRI done—that's before the rehab even began. The technology is there, we just have to get access to it and learn how to apply it to our specific needs. We now employ ultrasound, micro-current,

TENs, intramuscular stimulation, acupressure, manual manipulation, and cold laser, among other technology and techniques in the treatment of chronic head pain.

The treatment of chronic pain in the head and neck region is made more difficult by the close proximity of structures of our senses. The nose, ears, mouth, and eyes are very close together, and the different disorders causing pain that occur in each structure can easily overlap with one another. The expertise for pain control in the oral cavity and TM joint area belongs to the dental field. We are able to selectively bring the most effective treatment modality from dentistry to the equation. The goal is the same: we use dental appliances and techniques first to control and eliminate pain, and then further rehabilitation to eliminate any imbalances and restore health.

A cautionary word about medication use in these patients and in general: some medication deals specifically with an identifiable condition, such as the use of anticonvulsants in Trigeminal Neuralgia patients, is advisable. However, most pain control drugs such as opioids, anti-inflammatories, muscle relaxants, sedatives, etc., should be used on a very short-term basis. They are great in the initial phase of treatment, to reduce pain and relax the patients so normal healing response of the body can occur. When the body cannot overcome the injury process, long-term use of these medications will not help healing, and will only mask the symptoms at best. In fact, long-term use of some medication can hurt the body with their side effects, and some drugs such as opioids have serious addictive properties. Another common complication of long-term drug use is the rebound effect. In terms of pain, the medication overuse can actually become pain-producing, and the primary reason for its propagation.

Once the type of headache pain and extent of dental foundation imbalance is determined, treatment options are discussed. Historically, the treatments for headache pain included one or a combination of herbal remedies, stress-reduction exercises, massage, acupuncture, non-steroidal anti-inflammatory drugs (NSAID), narcotic pain relievers, anti-seizure medications, chiropractic adjustments, anti-depressants, or sedatives. Now, by using the combination of advanced dentistry techniques and sports rehabilitation-derived therapies used in treating dental force imbalances in dental headache care, we can reduce or eliminate the long-term use of medications and their side effects. This rehabilitative method resulted in dentists reporting 93 percent success rate in providing patients with real, lasting relief from their pain symptoms. The methods used control muscle force and force balance; restore proper function and range of motion, and change the way the brain perceives stimuli—so pain levels, dysfunction, and improper muscle activity return to normal. By balancing the muscles, joints, and teeth, and controlling the way the body feels pain in the head and neck areas, long-lasting pain relief can finally be achieved.

What this means is that because dentists are the primary healthcare practitioners capable of diagnosing problems both inside the mouth and the structures around the face and head, and since many of the pain conditions in this area refer pain from one area to another, making them more complex, dentists have the responsibility to diagnose and treat these chronic pain conditions. Therefore, dentists must be one of the first choices for patients who are seeking solutions to their chronic pain conditions.

Our professional mandate specifies that we have the proper training for diagnosing and treating conditions not just inside the oral cavity, but muscles, joints, and soft tissues of the head, neck, and jaw, and the nervous system associated with these tissues. More and more dentists are becoming serious about treating these life-altering conditions; you owe it to yourself to seek out a qualified dentist for your head pain today and get your life back.

TRACK 7:

NEW TECHNOLOGIES

My colleagues say I hold the record because I had braces four times. So my interest and vision is to find ways that will make getting your smile a better experience than mine was. What do I mean by "better"? Well, as a patient—yes, I know that was many years ago, but we won't go into that—my issues were that my mouth hurt, it took too long, and even though I ended up with straight teeth, I wasn't completely happy with my smile, even after all that painstaking work.

So I want to share with you some of the exciting technologies that are now available to help make your road to Rocking Your Smile easier and better than mine. As I am writing this in the last part of 2016, I am sure there are new technologies that will soon be released—I am even involved with consulting on a couple that are currently in development. But these are the latest and greatest at this time, and I believe if your orthodontist is using many of these, you can feel confident that you are in great hands and well on your way to your Rock Star Smile.

Digital Imaging

How many of you remember taking a picture with an actual camera? After the camera roll was full (usually no more than 36 images) you'd take out the film roll and drive down to the local photoshop or pharmacy. Then you would give them the roll and select the print type and paper size you wanted. Then you would have to return to pick them up in a week or so, only to find out that half of your family photos did not come out very well—someone blinked or wasn't looking at the camera, or (in my case) your finger was in the way.

Now, hardly anyone still uses the old film-based version of pictures. We have all gone digital. That means that the image is stored in small bits of information called pixels and stored on a computer. The computer can then put the pixels back together to re-create your image.

There are many advantages of using digital imaging. You can instantly see if your image is what you wanted (and make sure your finger is not in the way). You can enhance, modify, blend—all sorts of things the computer can help you do to get the image that you want. Digital images can also be more easily stored, categorized, and shared than their older version of print.

Digital imaging—photographs

As you are probably aware, this has been unanimously adopted into dentistry/orthodontics because it allows us to look at and discuss your teeth instantly, instead of the "waiting game" and having to return in a week.

Digital imaging—X-rays

Digital dental X-rays are making a huge difference in dental care. Initially, this technology took a little longer in development because of the size of the digital sensor and the cost to the dentist. Now, however, vast improvements have been made and most offices have adopted digital X-rays.

Digital imaging—3D cone beam

In orthodontics, we need additional views of your whole head so we can evaluate your skeletal growth and the development of your teeth and jaws. Dental imaging took a major leap forward at the beginning of the new millennium with a three-dimensional (3D) technology known as cone beam computed tomography ("tomo"–cut or slice; "graph"–picture). With cone beam computed tomography (CBCT), dentists can get amazingly detailed 3D views of the facial skeleton and teeth. Having a 3D CBCT image of you is like having your own holographic image. We can rotate it, look inside it, and now can even manipulate it to predict and design a plan to help you Rock Your Smile.

Digital Imaging–intraoral scanners

Have you ever had an impression or mold of your teeth? Was it a pleasurable and fun experience? Well, not for me. I still remember when I was in seventh grade. I had to go to my orthodontist to get a new retainer (I'm sure my "dog ate it"). I was already sweating and dreading the impression because I knew I was going to gag. Boy, did I ever–I even threw up. I was so embarrassed. Since then, there have been great improvements in the material used where it doesn't take as much and it sets up much quicker, so we rarely have this problem.

But what if I told you that you might never have to have an impression? That would be awesome, huh? As soon as I saw a digital scanner in the early 2000s and saw its potential to eliminate the need for even some of the impressions, I immediately got one. This would basically produce a digital impression of your teeth. There are other advantages similar to digital photos. It allows the doctor to evaluate if he likes the picture and the way it turned out immediately. It also has the ability to be stored on a computer, categorized, and shared with others without you having to take impressions all over again. I knew if I could keep from having to take impressions, then we all would win.

Space Age or Shape Memory Wires

I remember laying there in the orthodontic chair. It was time to change my wire. Oh no! That meant my orthodontist was going to take out a stiff stainless steel wire, then skillfully place the precise movements he thought my teeth needed. It would look like a piece of art. But then the assistant would have to force it in to my braces and use other wires to hold it in place. I could feel the pain (they called it "pressure") even before I got out of the chair.

So you can imagine how excited I was when I was in my orthodontic training and they came out with a new metal. A metal that could be used for these archwires call NiTiNOL. NiTiNOL is a Smart Shape Memory Alloy (SMA), meaning it remembers its shape. It stands for NI (Nickel), TI

(Titanium), N (Naval), O (Ordinance), and L (Laboratory). It was originally discovered in the NOL for missile tips and used by the space industry in satellites.

The material is used in orthodontics as wire to move the teeth. Once the SMA is placed in the mouth, its temperature rises to ambient body temperature. This causes the NiTiNOL to contract back to its original shape, applying a constant, light force to move the teeth. These SMA wires don't need to be retightened as often as conventional stainless steel wires, which distort immediately after they are tied into your braces. These SMA wires also use much lighter forces to move teeth. What does this mean to you? LESS PAIN!

NiTiNOL can be used for medical purposes, like knee replacements, and to reattach tendons to bones. It can also be used in glasses as frames, so that you can bend it and it will remember its shape before it was bent. It can be used many other ways as well.

Computerized individualized smile planning

Using new 3D intraoral scanning and computerized cone beam technology, your teeth can be simulated on the computer screen. A skilled orthodontist can then move your teeth to simulate what movements are possible and necessary to create the smile of your dreams. This way your smile is actually designed and planned, instead of the old-fashioned, traditional way of putting braces on and seeing what happens, modifying as you go and seeing where you end up.

Self-ligating brackets

Self-ligating braces are defined as "an orthodontic bracket which generally utilizes a permanently installed, moveable component to hold in the archwire." One of the most significant differences from conventional dental braces is the absence of the elastic ligature (bands or ties)—although we can apply some to your front braces for some fun, like red and green for Christmas or your school colors or your favorite team. Since these self-ligating braces use a slide mechanism, or door, to hold the archwire, the amount of pressure or force needed to move the teeth is greatly reduced. This means less pain. I don't know about you, but this I like!

Clear aligners

Many patients don't want to wear or can't wear braces on their teeth. In the middle of the year 2000, a company began to develop an option to move teeth and create your smile without using braces and wires. This was, as most of you know, Align Technology, the makers of Invisalign. It didn't work perfectly at the beginning, but with their commitment both in technology and financial investment, we now have a very good alternative to braces. Invisalign, or clear aligners, straighten your teeth using a custom-made series of aligners created for you and only you. These aligner trays are made of smooth, comfortable, and virtually invisible plastic that you wear over your teeth. They gradually and gently shift your teeth into place.

The advantages of aligner therapy (there are several other companies coming to market besides Invisalign) are trifold: one, they are virtually invisible; two, you can take them out to eat whatever you want and to better brush and floss; and three, because you don't have any brackets or wires, you eliminate a lot of the potential mouth sores.

Accelerated movements

Surgically assisted:

If you want your teeth straightened in less than a year, you might be a candidate for Periodontally Assisted Osteogenic Orthodontics (we use "PAOO," because that's a mouthful to say), sometimes called Wilckodontics (the two brothers that developed this technique are Tom and Bill Wilcko). This is an in-office procedure that causes the bone make-up to be changed and allows teeth to actually move faster through the bone. This is a great procedure for anyone that would also need some gum surgery. It just makes sense to speed up the whole thing. There are only two disadvantages: additional costs, and a procedure which will temporarily add more discomfort—but this won't last, and you can get your braces off in less than half the normal time.

Microperforations

A similar procedure is done using a specifically designed device (Propel) which will create these microperforations. It is less invasive than the previous procedure. It might be limited when compared to total movement of the PAOO technique, but it still does a very nice job of reducing the total treatment time until you are Rockin' Your Smile.

Micropulses

AcceleDent Aura speeds orthodontic treatment:

- Exclusive SoftPulse Technology applies precisely calibrated micropulses to gently accelerate the movement of your teeth as they are guided by your orthodontics.
- Safe acceleration of the bone remodeling process complements conventional orthodontic treatment.
- Clinically proven to move teeth up to 50 percent faster.

Part of the way that orthodontics works is by changing or remodeling the bones surrounding your teeth. As this remodeling process is accelerated, your teeth move more quickly. That's where AcceleDent comes in. By using tiny vibrations, or micropulses, SoftPulse Technology is designed to speed up bone remodeling, accelerating tooth movement.

3D printers

Have you ever seen plaster models? Have you ever made a mold of something and poured it full of Plaster of Paris? This process is similar to how dentistry has made models of your teeth for years. The drawbacks of this process are the following: you have to take impressions; there is possible distortion as the plaster sets; the model fractures in the middle of making an appliance. The ability to take a computerized model of your teeth and print it on one of the new 3D digital printers addresses these limitations: no impressions (when combined with one of the intraoral scanners); no distortion, they are very accurate, and the plastic model is very strong and would be difficult to fracture—but if it does, you can simply reprint the model, which saves you not having to take another impression.

Let me stress that these are the current technologies that help me deliver my vision—to reduce the amount of time it takes for your braces, to reduce the amount of soreness or discomfort you experience from your braces, and to improve the overall experience. I am sure, and hopeful, that there will be new techniques and technology for us to continue to improve upon these areas.

TRACK 8:

COMMON QUESTIONS

1. **What is orthodontics?**
   a. From the Greek "ortho" meaning straight and "odontos" for teeth, orthodontics is a specialty of dentistry aimed at the diagnostic, prevention and treatment of dento-facial anomalies and dental malpositions.
   b. The technical term to describe these problems is "malocclusion".
   c. Orthodontics is the branch of dentistry that specializes in the diagnosis, prevention, and treatment of dental and facial irregularities. The technical term for these problems is "malocclusion," which means "bad bite." The practice of orthodontics requires professional skill in the design, application, and control of corrective appliances, such as braces, to bring teeth, lips, and jaws into proper alignment, thus achieving facial balance.

2. **What is an orthodontist**
   a. An orthodontist is a dental specialist in the diagnosis, prevention, and treatment of dental and facial irregularities. Orthodontists must first attend college, then complete a four-year graduate dental program at a university-level dental school accredited by the American Dental Association (ADA). They must then complete an additional two- to three-year residency program of advanced dental education in orthodontics accredited by the ADA. Only dentists who have completed this advanced specialty education may become orthodontists.

3. **How do I know if my child needs ortho treatment**
   a. It can be very difficult to determine just by looking at your child. Many things cannot be seen without evaluating the growth and development of your childs teeth and jaws. We use a 3D imaging

machine that gives us a very clear picture of this as well as the ability to evaluate their airway. We suggest that you have you child's initial visit no later than age seven.

4. **What are the causes of malocclusions (crooked teeth)**

   a. Most malocclusions are inherited, and some are acquired. Inherited problems include crowding of teeth, too much space between teeth, extra teeth, congenitally missing teeth, and a wide range of discrepancies involving the jaws, teeth, and face. Acquired problems can be caused by trauma, thumb or finger sucking, airway obstruction by tonsils and adenoids, dental diseases, and premature loss of baby or adult teeth. Many of these problems affect not only the alignment of the teeth but facial development and appearance as well.

5. **What are the early signs of orthodontic problems**

   a. Although you may find it difficult to determine whether treatment is necessary, the following signs can help in prompting you to seek orthodontic advice: crowded or overlapping teeth; gaps between the teeth; poor alignment of front top teeth with bottom teeth; top front teeth that do not meet with the bottom teeth; and top front teeth that cover more than 50% of the bottom teeth. If you see any misalignment or shifting of the jaw, your child may have a skeletal problem that could require early orthodontic treatment.

6. **At what age should my child see an orthodontist**

   a. The American Association of Orthodontics recommends that your child be evaluated by age 7. We would recommend seeing your child no later than age 7. This will allow us evaluate for proper jaw growth, good tooth development, adequate airway. We can determine if treatment needs to start now or at a later time and inform you what to expect in the future.

7. **Am I too old**

   a. No, age is not a factor, only the health of your gums and bone which support your teeth. Currently about 35% of our orthodontic patients are adults (anyone older than 18yrs). We have had many of our adult patients in their 40's, 50's and 60's. Our oldest patient so far was an 84 yr old retired college professor. Many esthetic (invisible, clear) appliances make it now much more appealing for adults to Rock Their Smile.

8. **Can adults have braces**

   a. Age is not a factor in considering orthodontic treatment. Any adult in good general health with healthy gums and good bone support for the teeth is a good candidate for orthodontic treatment. About 35% of our orthodontic patients are adults, and that number is still growing!

9. **Is orthodontic treatment painful**

   a. Orthodontic treatment has improved dramatically. As a rule, braces make your teeth tender and sore for a few days. Our office takes extra steps to make your experience as comfortable as possible. We incorporate our exclusive Pain Reduce System to almost totally eliminate any discomfort from your braces.

10. **What are Phase 1 and Phase II treatments**

   a. Phase I treatment, if needed, usually starts between age 7 to 9. The goal of Phase I treatment is to improve any restricted airway problems, any skeletal growth discrepancies, and any tooth eruption problems. The goal of Phase 1 treatment is not necessarily to avoid full braces, but to avoid having to take out permanent teeth and to prevent having to have a jaw surgery.

   b. After a Phase 1 treatment, we will place your child in our Growth & Guidance Program. We will periodically see your child so we can determine when the best time will be to complete the final step to helping your child to Rock Their Smile!

11. Does everyone need a Phase 1 treatment?

   a. Not every child needs Phase I treatment. Only some children with certain bites require early treatment. Many will be able to move directly into our Growth and Guidance Program.

12. How long does a person wear braces?

   a. Treatment plans vary from six to roughly 30 months. Simpler cases can be finished more quickly. The overall average orthodontic treatment time is roughly 24 months. We have developed our exclusive OrthoBoost program that can reduce the time you are in braces by up to 50 percent. Our average is only a little over 14 months.

13. Is orthodontic care (braces) expensive?

   a. Orthodontic treatment can be expensive, but when you consider what the value is, it is actually a bargain. Not only will your teeth be much healthier, and easier to maintain, we know that people that have received proper orthodontic therapy will spend less in the future than they would have without orthodontic treatment. The benefit of a great smile, added confidence and better self esteem is priceless. We do offer our Interest Free Flex Payment Plan to help this life changing experience fit into your budget.

TRACK 9:

DENTAL SPECIALIST

Here is a brief description of the different dental specialists. If you need to see one, or one is involved with your case, you can reference this chapter and see what that means for you.

General Dentist (Primary Family Dentist) – the primary dental care providers for patients of all ages. They can treat you and your entire family and care for your overall oral health. This is crucial to your total health. Your general dentist takes responsibility for the diagnosis, treatment, and overall coordination of services to meet your oral health needs. If you need a specialized dental procedure performed, your general dentist may work with other dentists to make sure you get the care you need.

To become a general dentist, three or more years of undergraduate college education degree (typically with a strong science foundation) plus four years of dental school is required. After graduating, dentists must take a licensure examination which is required by the state in which they practice.

Cosmetic Dentist – normally a general dentist that specializes in cosmetic dental procedures: whitening, veneers, reshaping, etc.

Periodontist – a dentist who specializes in the prevention, diagnosis, and treatment of periodontal disease, and in the placement of dental implants. Periodontists are also experts in the treatment of oral inflammation. Periodontists receive extensive training in these areas, including three additional years of education beyond dental school. They are familiar with the latest techniques for diagnosing and treating periodontal disease, and are also trained in performing cosmetic periodontal procedures.

Endodontist – specialists in saving teeth, committed to helping you maintain your natural smile for a lifetime. They have at least two years of additional education to become experts in performing root canal treatments and diagnosing and treating tooth pain.

Oral Surgeon/Maxillofacial Surgeon – also known as OMS or OMFS. Dentists that specialize in treating many diseases, injuries, and defects in the head, neck, face, jaws, and the hard and soft tissues of the oral (mouth) and maxillofacial (jaws and face) region.

Orthodontist – a specialist who has undergone two to three years of special training in a dental school or college after they have graduated from dental school. The specialty deals primarily with the diagnosis, prevention, and correction of malpositioned teeth and the jaws.

Pediatric Dentist (Pedodontist) – specialists who have completed dental school and two additional years of residency training in dentistry for infants, children, teens, and children with special needs. Pediatric dentists are dedicated to the oral health of children from infancy through the teen years. They have the experience and qualifications to care for a child's teeth, gums, and mouth throughout the various stages of childhood.

Prosthodontist – this dental specialty requires an additional three years of training after graduating from dental school. Prosthodontists are primarily concerned with the restoration and replacement of lost or damaged teeth. Sometimes called the "architects of the smile," prosthodontists are highly trained specialists with a unique understanding of all the elements that go into a beautiful, functional, and natural-looking smile—not just the teeth, but also the gums, lips, and facial features.

Oral/Maxillofacial Pathologist – the specialty concerned with diagnosis and study of the causes and effects of diseases affecting the oral and maxillofacial region. It is sometimes considered to be a specialty of dentistry and pathology.

Oral/Maxillofacial Radiologist – also known as Dental and Maxillofacial Radiology. This specialty of dentistry must complete an additional two to four years of education after completing dental school. Oral radiology is concerned with performance and interpretation of diagnostic imaging used for examining the craniofacial, dental, and adjacent structures.

Implantologist – a dentist who specializes in implantology. This is not a recognized specialty by the American Dental Association.

TMJ Specialist – a dentist or specialist that has an emphasis in their practice on treating the pain and disorders associated with disorders of the temporal-mandibular joint (TMJ). It is not a recognized specialty of the American Dental Association.

Dental Hygienist – preventive oral health professionals who have graduated from an accredited dental hygiene program in an institution of higher education, usually an additional two to six years of college. Licensed in dental hygiene to provide educational, clinical, research, administrative, and therapeutic services supporting total health through the promotion of optimum oral health.

Dental Assistant – perform many tasks, ranging from providing patient care and taking X-rays to recordkeeping and scheduling appointments. Their duties vary by state and by the dentists' offices where they work. There are several possible paths to becoming a dental assistant. Some states require assistants to graduate from an accredited program and pass an exam. In other states, there are no formal educational requirements.

Dental Lab Technician – most dental laboratory technicians learn their craft on the job. They begin with simple tasks, such as pouring gypsum material into an impression, and progress to more complex procedures, such as making dentures, crowns, and bridges, or bending wires.

Becoming a fully trained technician requires an average of three to four years of experience on the job, depending upon the individual's aptitude and ambition, but it may take a few years more to become an accomplished technician.

Myofunctional Therapist/Speech Therapist – orofacial myology is a specialized professional discipline that evaluates and treats a variety of oral and facial (orofacial) muscle (myo-) postural and functional disorders and habit patterns that may disrupt normal dental development and also create cosmetic problems.

TRACK 10:

AT WHAT AGE DO TEETH COME IN?

I am including this section to help you understand the normal/average age that teeth normally come in. Remember, these are an *average*, so don't panic if you or your child is not exactly on this schedule. The exact age is not as important as the order, so that the teeth can all properly come into the mouth.

Primary/Baby teeth –

Primary Teeth

Upper Teeth	Erupt	Shed
Central Incisor	8-12 Months	6-7 Years
Lateral Incisor	9-13 Months	7-8 Years
Canine (Cuspid)	16-22 Months	10-12 Years
First Molar	13-19 Months	9-11 Years
Second Molar	25-33 Months	10-12 Years

Lower Teeth	Erupt	Shed
Second Molar	23-31 Months	10-12 Years
First Molar	14-18 Months	9-11 Years
Canine (Cuspid)	17-23 Months	9-12 Years
Lateral Incisor	10-16 Months	7-8 Years
Central Incisor	6-10 Months	6-7 Years

Permanent Teeth –

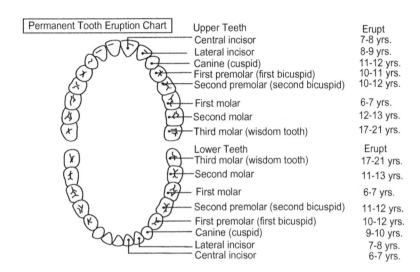

Permanent Tooth Eruption Chart		
Upper Teeth		**Erupt**
Central incisor		7-8 yrs.
Lateral incisor		8-9 yrs.
Canine (cuspid)		11-12 yrs.
First premolar (first bicuspid)		10-11 yrs.
Second premolar (second bicuspid)		10-12 yrs.
First molar		6-7 yrs.
Second molar		12-13 yrs.
Third molar (wisdom tooth)		17-21 yrs.
Lower Teeth		**Erupt**
Third molar (wisdom tooth)		17-21 yrs.
Second molar		11-13 yrs.
First molar		6-7 yrs.
Second premolar (second bicuspid)		11-12 yrs.
First premolar (first bicuspid)		10-12 yrs.
Canine (cuspid)		9-10 yrs.
Lateral incisor		7-8 yrs.
Central incisor		6-7 yrs.

TRACK 11:

DENTAL TERMS

A

Aesthetic – having to do with appearance and beauty, like a smile.

Amalgam – a silver filling.

B

Bicuspids/premolars – the teeth with two rounded points located between the eye teeth (canines/cuspids) and the molars.

Bleaching – the process of lightening or "whitening" the teeth to remove stains. The process usually involves a chemical oxidizing agent and sometimes uses heat.

Bonding – a technique to bind a filling or filling material to a tooth. Bonding materials may be used to repair chipped, cracked, misshapen, or discolored teeth, or to fill in a gap between teeth.

Bone loss – a decrease in the amount of bone that supports a tooth or implant.

Bridge – non-removable tooth replacements attached to adjoining natural teeth when one or more teeth are missing.

Bruxism – involuntary clenching or grinding of the teeth. Now being associated with sleep-airway issues. We see that when someone stops breathing at night, they grind their teeth to help open their airway and then take a breath.

C

Canines/cuspids – the teeth near the front of the mouth that come to a single point. Sometimes called the "eye teeth," or cuspids.

Caries – commonly used term for tooth decay.

Cavity – missing tooth structure. A cavity may be due to decay, erosion, or abrasion. If caused by caries, also can be referred to as a "carious lesion."

Centrals – the central incisor teeth. The front two teeth on both the upper and lower arches.

Composite – tooth-colored filling material used primarily for front teeth. Although cosmetically superior, it is generally less durable than other materials.

Cosmetics/cosmetic dentistry – any services provided by dentists solely for the purpose of improving your appearance, not your health.

Crown – a single, artificial tooth that fits over a real tooth that has been specially shaped. It can be used to replace missing tooth structure or reshape a malformed tooth. It can also fit over a dental implant.

Cusps – the pointed or rounded part of a tooth's biting surfaces.

Cuspids/canines – the teeth near the front of the mouth that come to a single point. Sometimes called the "eye teeth," or canines.

D

Decay – term for cavities. The decomposition of tooth structure.

Deciduous teeth – also called primary, or "baby" teeth. These are the first teeth a child gets.

Dental bridge – an appliance that fills the space left by missing teeth with artificial ones, held in place by attaching to natural teeth or implants.

Dental erosion – the thinning or wearing away of the hard coating of a tooth (the enamel).

Dentures – a set of artificial teeth. They can replace all of one's teeth (complete dentures) or a section of teeth (partial dentures).

Dry mouth – also called "xerostomia." A condition that results from an inadequate flow of saliva.

E

Enamel – the hard calcified tissue covering the dentin of the crown of the tooth.

Endodontics – treatment of the root and nerve of the tooth.

Esthetic – having to do with appearance and beauty, like a smile.

Extract – to pull or remove a tooth.

F

First molars/six-year molars – the molars (big teeth that you chew with) that are closest to the front of your mouth.

Floss – thick string used to remove food trapped between your teeth and remove bacteria that cannot be reached by brushing alone. It is usually made from nylon filaments or plastic monofilaments and may be treated with flavoring agents to make flossing more pleasant.

Fluoride – a mineral that helps prevent tooth decay (cavities).

Fluoride varnish – a liquid, containing fluoride, which is painted onto the teeth and then hardens. This provides a temporary protective shield.

G

Gingival – things having to do with your gums.

Gingivitis – inflammation (or infection) of the gum tissue without loss of connective tissue.

Gingival graft – see "graft."

Graft – a gingival graft, also called "gum graft" or "periodontal plastic surgery." This is a generic name for any of a number of periodontal surgical procedures in which the gum tissue is grafted. The aim may be to cover exposed root surfaces, or merely to augment the band of keratinized tissue.

Gum disease – a disease that may cause gums to be red, swollen, and bleed easily. If it is not treated, gum disease can get worse and can lead to bone loss and therefore compromise the long-term health of your teeth. It is also called "gingivitis," or "periodontal disease," depending on the severity.

H

I

Impacted tooth – a tooth beneath the gum tissue that lies against another tooth, under bone or soft tissue, which is unlikely to grow out on its own.

Implant – an artificial tooth root that dentists put in the jaw bone. The dentist can put an artificial tooth (or crown) on the implant, or the implant can also be used to hold a bridge or even dentures in place.

Incisors – the front four teeth (including the central and lateral incisors) in both the upper and lower jaws.

Intraoral – having to do with inside the mouth.

J

Jaw – a common name for either the maxilla (upper jaw) or mandible (lower jaw).

K

L

Laser – an instrument that produces a very narrow, intense beam of light energy. When laser light comes in contact with tissue, it causes a reaction. The light produced by the laser can remove or shape tissue. In dentistry they are commonly used for the following: to treat gum disease; to re-contour the shape of gum tissue; tooth whitening; to improve healing of canker sores and ulcers; or to expose impacted teeth.

Laterals – lateral incisors. The teeth right next to the front two teeth (central incisors) on both the upper and lower jaws.

M

Malocclusion – a term used to describe teeth that don't line up correctly in the mouth. They may be too far apart, crooked, or may not come together correctly when you bite together.

Molars – the large teeth in the back of your mouth. We use our molars to chew food. These teeth have a broad chewing surface that is used for grinding food.

N

Nursing Bottle Syndrome – severe decay in baby teeth due to sleeping with a bottle of milk or juice. The drink's natural sugars combine with bacteria in the mouth.

O

Oral hygiene – activities you do to keep your mouth clean. These include brushing your teeth, cheeks, tongue, and oral appliances (retainers, dentures, etc.). They also can include using dental floss, a water pic, mouthwash, and having a dentist or dental hygienist clean your teeth.

Orthodontic treatment – used to make teeth line up correctly. Also see "malocclusion." Braces are one kind of orthodontic treatment. Clear aligners are another.

Overdenture – a prosthetic device (denture) that is supported by implants or the roots of at least two natural teeth to provide better stability for the denture.

P

Pediatric dentist – a dental specialty devoted to the treatment of children, from birth through adolescence.

Periapical – the area surrounding the end of a tooth root.

Periapical X-ray – the small X-ray taken of a tooth or teeth to evaluate the health of the teeth and surrounding bone.

Peri-implantitis – an infection that develops around an implant. It can cause bone loss, resulting in possible loss of the implant.

Periodontal disease – more commonly known as "gum disease," it is caused by plaque. When the plaque is not removed, it can cause your gums to pull away from your teeth. Your gums may also become inflamed (red and swollen) and bleed easily.

Periodontitis – a severe form of gum disease which can lead to tooth loss.

Plaque – a soft, sticky, thick layer of bacteria that forms on your teeth. It can easily be removed with good brushing and flossing techniques.

Post and Core – an anchor placed in the tooth root following a root canal to strengthen the tooth and help hold a crown in place.

Pontic – the portion of a dental bridge that replaces a missing tooth. In orthodontics, a pontic is a plastic tooth that is attached to the wire to simulate a tooth that is missing.

Premolars/bicuspids – the teeth with two rounded points located between the eye teeth (canines/cuspids) and the molars.

Primary teeth – the first set of teeth that you get when you are a child. These are also called "baby teeth."

Prophylaxis – removal of plaque, calculus (tartar), and stains from the tooth structures. Usually called a "prophy," or teeth cleaning. This procedure is performed in the dental office.

Prophy – a cleaning or polishing of your teeth. This is normally done in the dental office.

Prosthodontics – replacement of missing teeth with artificial materials, such as a bridge or denture.

Pulp – the blood supply and nerves that run up the middle of each tooth.

Q

Quadrant – one of the four equal sections into which the dental arches can be divided. It begins at the midline, or middle of your front teeth, and extends to the last tooth on that side. So you have the upper-right, upper-left, lower-right, and lower-left.

R

Radiograph – a picture of the bones or teeth inside the body. Also called an "X-ray."

Recede – when the gums pull away from the teeth. It can also be called "recession."

Recession – when you gums pull away from the tooth. It can look like your teeth are getting longer, but it is actually that your gums are shrinking down toward the bottom of the tooth. This can also cause some root sensitivity, especially to cold.

Restorations – replacement of missing or damaged tooth structure with artificial materials, such as fillings, crowns, etc.

Retainer – a device used to stabilize teeth following orthodontic treatment.

Root canal treatment – a dental treatment for a tooth infection that has progressed far enough that the infection is now near the blood supply of the tooth. During a root canal, the blood and nerve supply that run down the middle of the tooth are removed. After that, the tooth is usually filled with a material and sealed, or is specially shaped and covered with an artificial tooth (a crown).

S

Sealant – a thick plastic coating that can be put on the tops of molars and premolars (the big teeth in the back of your mouth). Sealants get hard and keep food from getting packed in the deep surfaces of these teeth. They help to prevent cavities.

Sinuses – the spaces in the bones of your face, located in the forehead and on either side of the nose.

Sjogren's syndrome – an illness in which the immune system attacks the body's own cells by mistake. It mainly causes dry mouth and dry eyes, but can affect other areas of the body like the joints.

Staining – discoloration of tooth surfaces. This can happen as a result of injury, genetics, smoking, certain medications, drinking of coffee or tea, but is ultimately a part of aging.

T

Temporomandibular joint disorders (TMJ) – problems in your jaw joints that can cause popping, clicking sounds. It can cause your jaw to feel "locked" and can result in pain in the joints, ears, and even present as headaches.

Tooth decay – a hole in the tooth caused by the acid in the plaque. A more common name is "cavity."

Tooth extraction – the removal of a tooth from the bone socket and surrounding gums.

Topical – refers to medications that are applied to the surface of the body. Usually used in dentistry to provide some temporary numbness in the localized area.

U

Unerupted – a tooth that has not pushed through the gum line.

V

Veneer – thin, custom-made shells crafted of tooth-colored materials designed to cover the front sides of teeth.

W

Wear/attrition – the loss of normal tooth structure, caused either by excess force or chemical.

Whitening – any process that will make teeth appear whiter. It can be achieved with a bleaching or non-bleaching product. Whitening options range from in-office procedures, professional "take-home" materials, or over-the-counter products (such as whitening toothpastes).

Wisdom teeth – the last teeth to come in during young adulthood. Also called "third molars." The majority of our US population do not have room for these teeth to properly grow into the mouth, and therefore are normally removed by an oral surgeon.

X

Xerostomia – decreased salivary secretion (spit) that produces a dry and sometimes burning sensation. Also called "dry mouth."

X-ray – see "radiograph."

Y

Z

TRACK 12:

ORTHODONTIC TERMS

A

Alginate – a plaster-like compound used to take impressions. It might taste awful, but it is safe.

Aligners – clear aligners are an alternative to traditional braces and are designed to help guide teeth into their proper position. Similar to braces, clear aligners use a gradual force to control tooth movement, but without metal wires or brackets.

Ankylosed – Dental Ankylosis is an abnormal dental condition where there is a solid fixation of a tooth from a fusion of the root to the bone. Normally, around the roots of our teeth, there is gum tissue that is called the "periodontal ligament." Dental Ankylosis can occur with primary (baby) teeth and permanent (adult) teeth. It is more common in primary teeth than permanent teeth.

Archwires – the wire that attaches to your braces. It is called an "archwire" because your top teeth comprise your top arch, and your bottom teeth comprise your bottom arch. An archwire is like the engine that guides and moves your teeth. Without an archwire to connect your braces, you would just be wearing braces for fun and your teeth would never move! Archwires come in different sizes and have different material compositions.

Asymmetrical – having parts that fail to corresponde to one another in shape, size, or arrangement. Lacking symmetry.

B

Band – a metal ring to which brackets or other attachments can be connected. Bands are typically used on the back teeth.

Braces – today's orthodontics offer more kinds of braces than ever before. Check out your options:

- **Metal braces/Traditional braces** – the metal <u>brackets</u> and wires that most people picture when they hear the word "braces." However, modern brackets are smaller and less noticeable than the notorious "metal-mouth" braces many adults remember. Plus, new heat-activated <u>archwires</u> use your body heat to help teeth move more quickly and less painfully than in the past.
- **Ceramic Braces** – the same size and shape as metal braces, except that they have tooth-colored or clear <u>brackets</u> that blend in to teeth. Some even use tooth-colored wires to be even less noticeable.
- **Lingual Braces** – the same as traditional metal braces, except that the <u>brackets</u> and wires are placed on the inside of teeth.
- **Clear Aligners** – Invisalign consists of a series of eighteen to thirty custom-made, mouth guard–like clear plastic aligners. The aligners are removable and are replaced every two weeks.

Brackets – part of braces (see different types listed in "braces"). These are usually attached or bonded to your teeth and serve as "handles" that give the orthodontist something to hold on to and guide the tooth using the archwires.

C

Class I malocclusion – a malocclusion where your upper and lower teeth are close to fitting together.

Class II malocclusion – a malocclusion where your upper teeth stick out too far past your lower teeth. This increases the possibility of you chipping or banging your front teeth. Sometimes teased as "buck teeth."

Class III malocclusion/underbite – a malocclusion where your lower teeth stick out too far past your upper teeth. This is sometimes teased as "bulldog" or "looking mean."

Continuous/elastic chain/power chain – a group of the little color rubber bands hooked together. Looks like a chain. It is used to stretch across the teeth.

Congenitally missing teeth - missing of one or more teeth from birth is perhaps our most common congenital malformation. More than 20 percent of us lack one or more wisdom teeth (third molars). More than 5 percent of us lack one or more second premolars or upper second (lateral) incisors. Lack of a large amount of teeth, though, is much more rare.

Crossbite – a malocclusion where some of your upper teeth are inside of your lower teeth.

Crowding – misaligned teeth can occur as teeth develop, or from childhood habits such as thumb sucking. The most common cause is when the jaw is too small compared with the size of the teeth. In addition to misaligned teeth, symptoms may include discomfort or difficulty while chewing.

D

Deep bite – where your upper front teeth cover too much of your lower front teeth. They should only cover approximately 25 percent of your lower teeth.

Diastema – a space between two of your teeth.

E

Elastics/rubber bands – used to adjust bite and jaw position. These are connected to the brackets with hooks, often connecting the top tooth bracket with the bottom tooth bracket to help adjust the position of the teeth in the mouth and the position of the jaw. Interarch rubber bands help to ensure that your child's teeth will line up properly. These must be removed during meals as well as when cleaning teeth and orthodontic brackets. In addition, they are typically replaced daily because of the wear they endure. Not every child who gets braces will need rubber bands, as it depends on the child's existing jaw alignment and what the orthodontist recommends to the patient.

Elastic tie(s)/O-tie/elastomer – a small rubber tie that fits around the bracket and helps secure the archwire. O-ties come in many colors.

Elastic chain/power chain – made of the same material as the elastic ties. The elastics form a continuous chain that can be used instead of the elastics. Elastic chain is used to close gaps between teeth.

Elastomers/elastic tie(s)/O-tie – a small rubber tie that fits around the bracket and helps secure the archwire. O-ties come in many colors.

Esthetic gingival re-contouring – if your gums rest too low or too high on your teeth and you are unhappy with your smile, you may be a candidate for gum contouring surgery. Also called "gum reshaping" or "tissue sculpting," this cosmetic dental procedure can even out an uneven gum line and give you a smile you can be proud of.

Esthetic tooth re-contouring – re-contouring or reshaping the teeth (also called "odontoplasty," "enameloplasty," "stripping," or "slenderizing") is a procedure in which small amounts of tooth enamel are removed to change a tooth's length, shape, or surface. The procedure is usually done to improve appearance by creating more harmony or balance in the look of the smile. Re-contouring is the most conservative cosmetic treatment. It is a quick and painless procedure whose results can be seen immediately.

Expander – a palatal expander, also known as a rapid palatal expander, rapid maxillary expansion appliance, palate expander, orthodontic expander, Haas, or Hyrax, is used to widen the upper jaw (maxilla) so that the bottom and upper teeth will fit together better.

Exposure/tooth exposure – needed when you have a tooth that is impacted, or still covered by either bond, gum tissue, or both. The tooth can be exposed by having the gum and/or bone removed enough to allow the tooth to erupt into the mouth. This can often be done today using a small laser. Usually we will bond a small bracket or attachment to your tooth, so we can begin to move your tooth into its proper position.

Extrusion – tooth movement in the direction of eruption. Natural extrusion: teeth grow until they touch the opposing teeth.

F

Forsus Spring – spring-coil rods that are permanently attached to the braces. These rods are used to correct short lower jaws, or those not wearing elastics.

Frenectomy – also known as a "frenulectomy." The removal of a frenulum, a small fold of tissue that prevents an organ in the body from moving too far. Done mostly for orthodontic purposes, a frenectomy is either performed inside the middle of the upper lip, which is called "labial frenectomy," or under the tongue, called "lingual frenectomy." Frenectomy is a very common dental procedure that is performed on infants, children, and adults. A similar procedure, "frenulotomy," is where a tight frenulum may be relieved by making an incision in the tight tissue.

Frenulectomy – see "frenectomy."

Full orthodontic treatment – getting braces.

G

Gingival display/excessive gingival display – description of the amount of gingiva that you show when you smile. It can affect the esthetics of your smile if/when excessive.

H

Hawley Retainer – this includes a metal wire that typically surrounds the six anterior teeth and keeps them in place. Named for its inventor, Dr. Charles A. Hawley, the labial wire, or Hawley bow, incorporates two omega loops for adjustment. It is anchored in an acrylic arch that sits in the palate (roof of the mouth). The advantage of this type of retainer is that the metal wires can be adjusted to finish treatment and continue minor movement of the anterior teeth as needed. With the improvement in the clear retainers, the Hawley Retainer has limited use right now.

Hook – an attachment for elastics. Hooks can be connected to brackets and bands or attached to archwires.

I

Impacted tooth – a tooth beneath the gum tissue that lies against another tooth, under bone or soft tissue, which is unlikely to grow out on its own.

Interproximal stripping – polishing the enamel of the tooth. This is used to adjust the tooth size and keep it in proper fit with the rest of your teeth.

Intrusion – movement of the tooth back into the bone.

Invisible braces/clear braces/Invisalign – straightening your teeth with either clear braces bonded to your teeth or using removal aligners (Invisalign).

IPR/striping – See "interproximal reduction"

Interproximal reduction (IPR) – also called interproximal enamel reduction, slenderizing, air rotor stripping (ARS), or reproximation. The practice of mechanically removing enamel from between the teeth to achieve orthodontic ends, such as to correct crowding, or reshape the contact area between neighboring teeth.

J

Jaw surgery – see "surgical correction."

K

K-hooks – a thin wire used to add a hook onto a bracket. Primarily used when you need to wear elastics, if your bracket doesn't already have a hook on it.

L

Ligature tie – a thin wire used to secure the archwire to the bracket.

Lingual appliances – orthodontic appliances fixed to the inside of your teeth. These are sometimes called "invisible" and/or "esthetic" braces.

Lingual arch – an orthodontic holding appliance for the lower arch. It is used to help hold space so the permanent teeth can erupt.

Lingual retainers – a bonded retainer. It is glued behind all of the lower front teeth.

M

Malocclusion – a misalignment or incorrect relation between the teeth of the two dental arches when they approach each other as the jaws close. Correction of malocclusion may reduce risk of tooth decay and help relieve excessive pressure on the temporomandibular joint (TMJ). Orthodontic treatment is also used to align for aesthetic reasons.

N

Nickel Titanium – see "NiTi."

NiTi (nickel titanium) archwires – Niti, Nitinol, Nickel Titanium alloy discovered in the late 1950s by the US Naval Ordinance Laboratory (hence the "NOL" portion of the name NiTiNOL). Depending upon the heat-treat history, nitinol has the ability to exhibit either superelastic properties or shape memory characteristics.

NiTiNOL – see "NiTi."

O

Open bite – a term used to describe when the upper and lower teeth are unable to make physical contact with each other when the jaws are closed.

In an ideal bite, the upper teeth should slightly overlap lower teeth in the vertical dimension by about 25 percent.

An open bite can be a "skeletal open bite," meaning that the jaw bones are growing away from each other. It can also be a developmental open bite—thumb sucking, lip sucking, or tongue thrusting.

Orthognathic surgery – see "surgical correction."

O-tie/elastic tie/elastomer – a small rubber tie that fits around the bracket and helps secure the archwire. O-ties come in many colors.

Overbite/overjet – most commonly described as a condition where the upper front teeth are significantly forward or in front of the lower front teeth. A severe overbite can lead to an increased likelihood of trauma to the upper front teeth from a fall or injury, and it can also make it difficult to bite into some foods. Your orthodontist or dentist might use this term to describe how much your upper teeth overlap your lower teeth vertically.

Overjet – see "overbite."

P

Palatal expander – also known as a rapid palatal expander, rapid maxillary expansion appliance, palate expander, orthodontic expander, Haas, or Hyrax. Used to widen the upper jaw (maxilla) so that the bottom and upper teeth will fit together better.

Phase I – early interceptive treatment. An orthodontic treatment (i.e., expansion and/or partial braces) that is done before all of the permanent teeth have erupted, and often occurs between the ages of five and eleven. The goal of Phase I treatment is to correct skeletal growth, create and hold adequate space for all permanents to erupt, and to make sure your child has a good airway.

Phase II – complete set of braces or aligners after your child has had a Phase I treatment. This is used to finish the orthodontic treatment.

Power chain/elastic chain – made of the same material as the O-ties. The elastics form a continuous chain that can be used instead of the elastics. Power chain is used to close gaps between teeth.

Q

R

Rapid palatal expander – also known as a palatal expander, rapid maxillary expansion appliance, palate expander, orthodontic expander, Haas, or Hyrax. Used to widen the upper jaw (maxilla) so that the bottom and upper teeth will fit together better.

Retainers – are custom-made devices, usually made of clear plastic, sometimes of wire and acrylic, and sometimes a wire bonded to the inside of your teeth. Retainers are designed to hold teeth in position after orthodontic tooth movement.

Retained primary teeth – it is not uncommon for primary or baby teeth to be retained past the normal time for them to fall out. This is most commonly caused by the permanent or adult teeth under them missing part of the root of the baby tooth so it can't get loose. The other common reason is if the permanent tooth is congenitally (or naturally) missing, therefore the baby tooth doesn't resorb and fall out like normal.

Rubber bands – an important part of the orthodontic treatment. They provide the connective force necessary to move the teeth and jaw into the proper alignment. Rubber bands are used to adjust bite and jaw position. These are connected to the brackets with hooks, often connecting the top tooth bracket with the bottom tooth bracket to help adjust the position of the teeth in the mouth and the position of the jaw. Rubber bands help to ensure that your child's teeth will line up properly.

S

Separator/spacer – a rubber ring slightly larger than an Elastic-tie that is placed in-between two teeth. The purpose of separators is to create space for bands. A separator can also be a wire separator, if needed.

Spacer/separator – a rubber ring slightly larger than an O-tie that is placed in-between two teeth. The purpose of separators is to create space for bands. A spacer can also be a wire separator, if needed.

Spacing – when your teeth have spaces between them. They should have contact with their neighbors, adjacent teeth, on both sides. This can be an esthetic concern but also a health concern for the teeth and the supporting gums and bone.

Striping/IPR – see "interproximal reduction."

Surgical correction/jaw surgery/orthognathic surgery – surgery to correct conditions of the jaw and face related to structure, growth, sleep apnea, TMJ disorders, malocclusion problems owing to skeletal disharmonies, or other orthodontic problems that cannot be easily treated with braces. Originally coined by Harold Hargis, it is also used in treatment of congenital conditions like cleft palate. Bones can be cut and realigned, then held in place with either screws or plates. Orthognathic surgery can also be referred to as corrective jaw surgery.

Symmetrical/symmetry – a balance between the left and right side, usually used in evaluating both sides of your face or your smile.

T

Third (3rd) molars/wisdom teeth – one of the three molars per quadrant of the human mouth. It is the most posterior (farther back) of the three. Wisdom teeth generally erupt between the ages of 17 and 25. Most humans today do not have adequate room for these to erupt; therefore, it is normally recommended that these be removed, or extracted.

U

V

W

Wire tie – a thin wire used to secure the archwire to the bracket.

Wires – see "archwires."

Wisdom teeth – see "third (3rd) molars."

X

Y

Z

TRACK 13:

PARTS OF BRACES

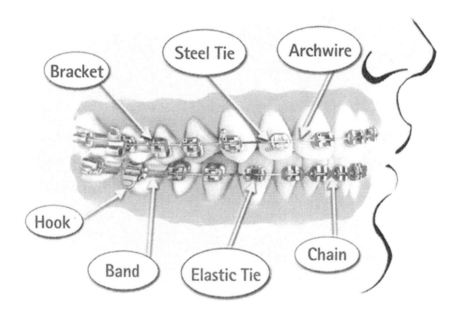

TRACK 14:

PATIENT COMMENTS

"As always, the staff at Whitlock were all excellent and very friendly and professional all at once. My daughter, being told that the time has come finally for braces, was excited and nervous all at once, but her comfort with the staff and Dr. Whitlock put her at ease. Thanks to Dr. Whitlock and all the staff there and for all you do to make your patients feel at ease!"

"At 63 years of age, my case was a challenge to say the least. But Dr. Whitlock and his incredible staff met the challenge beyond expectations—and always with warm smiles and caring concern for my comfort and satisfaction! My sincere thanks to all."

"My son recently had his braces removed; his smile is amazing and being able to share this smile with confidence has made a huge impact on his self-esteem. Dr. Whitlock and his staff go over and beyond the call of duty for each person during and after treatment. I cannot put into words my appreciation as a mom. Thank you!"

"Dr. Whitlock, I am so pleased every time I bring both kids in for their appointments, from the time I walk in, with the friendly welcome, to just knowing our names each time we come—it is too nice! Both kids really like coming, which is also a big play! I cannot think of one thing I would change. Thank you for always making our trip to the orthodontist a stress-free and pleasant one."

"Experience was great. Staff was informative and answered all my questions. Wait time was short and appointment was quick."

"Had Invisalign for only six months!!! Great experience!! This office is Awesome!!"

"Dr. Whitlock and team are by far the best. Not only did they go above and beyond to make my daughter feel comfortable, they are exceptionally nice. I had to bring my three-year-old with me to an appointment and everyone was so good to her. I will definitely recommend Dr. Whitlock to anyone that is looking for an orthodontist. Thank you, Dr. Whitlock and team, for all that you do. You are amazing!!"

"My daughter has had Invisalign for several months now. Her teeth are noticeably straighter and the results have been amazing. The staff at Whitlock Ortho are friendly and enthusiastic. I am very happy we chose Whitlock for her orthodontic needs."

"Best decision I ever made. Love the way my smile looks after wearing braces for just a year. Now wearing retainers. Was one of the best decisions I ever made. Everyone at Dr. Whitlock's office is great. I appreciate the excellent care I have received."

"I really enjoyed my experience here at Whitlock Orthodontics! The staff is wonderful and I'm extremely happy with the outcome. I couldn't be more grateful to have such a great smile and to meet such amazing people! I would recommend them to anyone who wants that perfect smile. Thank you all so much!"

BONUS TRACK #1: SUMMARY

"WHAT DO I LOOK FOR?"

I created this summary list to assist you when looking for an orthodontist. Evaluate and score the doctor and office that you visit to help compare what is actually important.

1. Find a doctor and a team with compassion. You want to find a team that treats you the same way they would treat a member of their own family.

2. Find a doctor and team that evaluates you and treats you and your total body health. Some orthodontists/dentists might treat your teeth, but not as a part of your total health.

   a. Someone that will evaluate and treat your airway.

   b. Someone that will evaluate and treat your headaches and migraines.

   c. Someone that will evaluate your teeth and the surrounding bone and make sure that the roots of your teeth are in the bone.

   d. Someone that evaluates your lip support, and the tooth position that improves your lip support to maintain a more youthful appearance.

3. Find a doctor with excellent reviews and evaluations. It is important to know how both patients and other professionals feel about the treatment that your doctor's office provides. Check out their Google reviews, Facebook comments, etc.

4. Find a doctor that invests in you and the quality of care they provide. Evaluate whether they are continuing to expand, explore, and improve the service that they provide, versus still practicing the way they did when they got out of school. Do they attend continuing education courses? Do they invest in new technologies that improve the quality of your treatment experience?

5. Find a doctor that offers financial flexibility. Not necessarily the cheapest, because if they are investing in you and the quality of care they provide, they can't be the cheapest. But do they offer some financing options to help you work this into your monthly budget?

BONUS TRACK #2:

WHY WHITLOCK ORTHO?

Because of my past experience (having braces four times) and my passion to create a better overall experience, we at Whitlock Orthodontics strive to provide the best place for you to get the smile of your dreams. Here are some ways that make us the best place for you to Rock Your Smile:

1. **Whitlock Ortho's** *OrthoBoost Program* - because I understand and appreciate the desire to get your smile without having braces on for years and years, I have put together an exclusive program for you that can reduce your time in treatment by up to 40 percent when compared to traditional orthodontic therapy.

2. **Whitlock Ortho's** *Pain Reduce System* - because I have experienced having my braces tightened many times before, I have put together our Pain Reduce System as a gift for you. It can reduce any pain and/or discomfort by nearly 80 percent.

3. **Customized Treatment Plan** - every orthodontic treatment is unique, just like every smile is equally as unique. Upon your first visit, we will design and tailor make the ultimate customized treatment plan built for your specific smile!

4. **Whitlock Ortho's** *Ortho Taxi* - as a courtesy to you, and understanding how difficult it can be to get your kid to their appointment, we developed our Ortho Taxi service. We have our customized Whitlock Ortho Hummer come pick up your kid from area schools, bring them to their appointments, and then return them back to school.

5. **Whitlock Ortho's** *3D Airway Screening* - it's true that right now your or your child's airway may be partially blocked! It's far more common than most people would expect, and specially trained orthodontists are considered among the world's top experts in airway treatment.

6. **Whitlock Ortho's** *Head and Neck Pain Vulnerability Assessment* – the next time you experience a headache or stiff neck, it may very possibly be happening for reasons that are preventable.

7. **Whitlock Ortho's** *Retainers For Life Program* – once your orthodontic treatment is complete, your retainer will help keep your new Rock Star Smile in perfect alignment. Over the course of the next several years, retainers need to be replaced, which can cost as much as $400 each time. With our Retainers For Life program, you'll never spend a dime to replace your worn-out retainer!

8. **Whitlock Ortho's** *Interest-Free Flex Payment Plan* – if you have looked at receiving orthodontic treatment in the past, then you know that the payment options are narrow and often times not accommodating to your budget. With the Whitlock Ortho Interest Free FlexPay System, you'll not only receive zero percent interest but you will have your investment custom tailored to fit your specific needs!

BONUS TRACK #3:

BEFORE AND AFTER PICS

Patient: AU

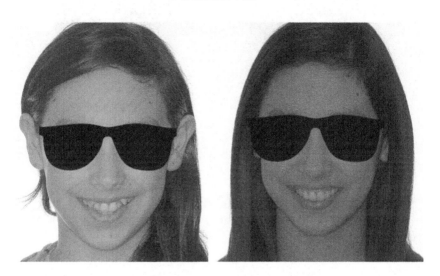

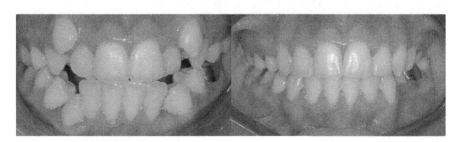

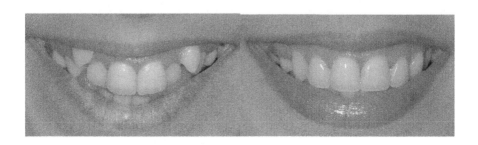

Patient: BR

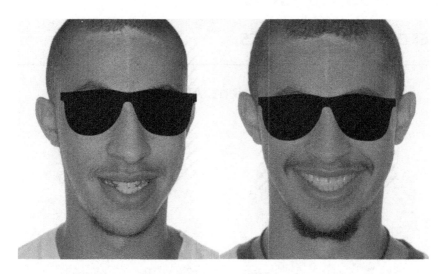

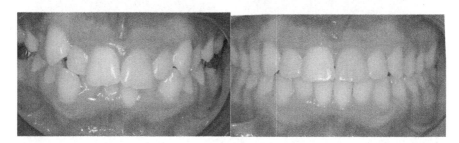

Patient: LG

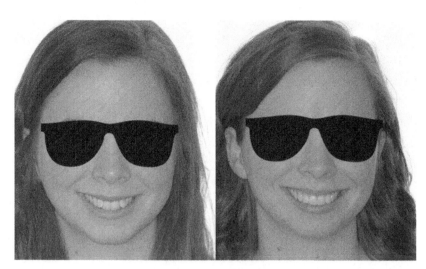

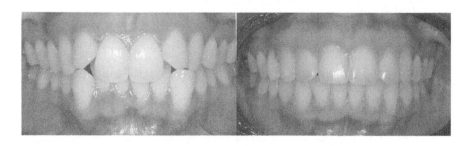

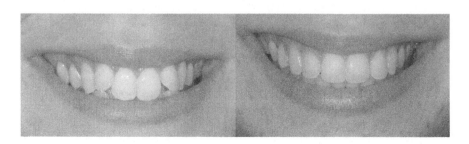

Patient: SP

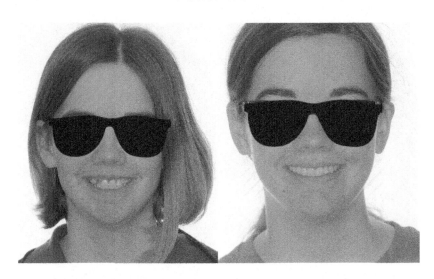

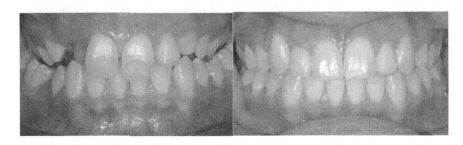

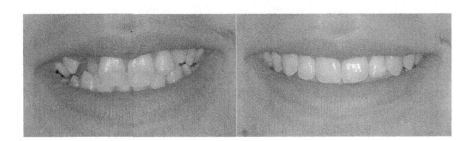

Patient: VH

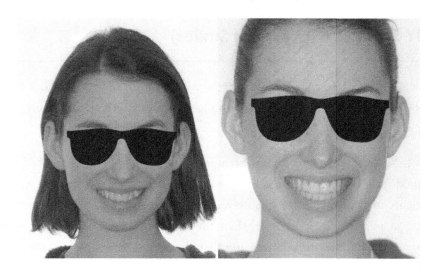

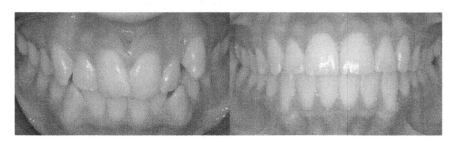

BONUS TRACK #4:

DIY SMILE (Do It Yourself Smiles)

As we come to the end of this book, there is still a lot to be said about DIY (Do It Yourself) orthodontics, so I thought it would be best to address this topic.

Do It Yourself orthodontics has been around for many years. Several of my orthodontic faculty members shared with us things that they would instruct patients to help do things themselves—using a tongue blade to push teeth, using a popsicle stick to strengthen the lip muscle, etc. These were still "prescribed" by the orthodontist and then monitored on follow-up visits.

Do It Yourself has recently exploded with access to things like YouTube and Vimeo and Google. Now, anyone can share their experience and knowledge on anything. Many times, these can be very helpful. I have used these tools myself—how do I get my computer to restart, how to clean my grill, how to fix my car fob (keyless remote) or start my car without it, etc. These are all mechanical techniques that don't require a proper, professional diagnosis. None of these involve potential irreparable damage to a human being. So when people started sharing a few helpful items on social media sites, many of their friends and contacts benefitted from it.

Recently a company started marketing a product of direct-to-consumer aligners—close to a DIY product—which does not involve a doctor seeing you. They are marketing it as "cutting out the middle man." Well, I don't consider your doctor the "middle man" in anything. Totally different than you shopping on line, buying direct from the manufacturer—this would be where you would be truly "cutting out the middle man."

The founders of this company have previously taken hearing aids and contact lenses direct to consumers and so think this is the same thing. The difference is that if you are going in for a hearing check or an eye exam, you should be evaluated by a doctor. The doctor exams you, diagnoses your situation and writes a prescription for treatment of your situation, usually for a device or a product. The difference in this new orthodontic approach is that you take a couple of pictures and the lab does a simulation of your teeth correction (limited to minor movements) and a dentist/orthodontist might approve that setup. Although on average, it has been reported that they spend only about two or three minutes reviewing a case and are only compensated if they *approve* a case. *But* the doctor has not evaluated you, your teeth, etc., and then individualized your treatment plan.

So when this company was being formed, I was approached with their vision and asked to join their advisory board. I agreed to join so that I could help protect patients as we addressed this need to make orthodontic alignment and treatment more accessible to some patients. At first, they agreed and only treated minor movements and required that proper records and clinical evaluation were done prior to initiating orthodontic evaluation. I was in agreement with this type of approach. But as the company has continued the need to grow and reach other patients, they have dropped the requirement of proper evaluation from a dentist or orthodontist. ***Just three clinical photos.*** Many of the cases that I was being ask to approve had obvious health-related issues that if left untreated or addressed could cause more harm to the patient's health and often end up costing the patient more money.

The difference between clear aligner therapy and contact lenses is that a contact lens is a product. Once you receive the proper evaluation and diagnosis of what your eye-correction need is, the eye doctor writes a prescription of lens correction for glasses, contacts, etc. Orthodontic aligners are not simply a "product," but a series of therapeutic devices. Like surgical instruments: just because you might be able to go out and buy a surgical scalpel and can find an instructional video doesn't mean you should perform your own surgery.

Don't misunderstand me, I do believe this has a place. Not currently truly DIY, but a modified delivery system that is prescribed and monitored by your local orthodontist is very helpful.

Anyone can make an aligner. It is simply a piece of plastic that is adapted to your model of your teeth. To be active, it has built-in tooth movements, which may or may not be possible or healthy for you.

So, it is true that anyone can make an "aligner," just like everyone can follow a recipe. But the treatment might not always turn out to be perfect or the best, just like with a recipe—there are variables that a master chef is aware of, variables like oven temperature, altitude, fresh ingredients versus frozen, etc. The meal might taste OK—if you didn't know any different. So you need to involve a doctor to make sure you don't hurt yourself or your teeth and end up with a worse situation.

And when you all but eliminate the doctor from the treatment planning and actual treatment process, you are eliminating many of the safeguards that ensure you are properly treated. Remember, all doctors swear the whole "do no harm" oath thing. CEOs do not. I follow the mantra that my DR. actually stands for "Do Right."

So please consult your local orthodontist and ask them about an "at-home version" that they might be able to offer you, reducing your number of office visits, maybe some digital monitoring, but which would have a thorough professional evaluation from the beginning. You would have someone there with you throughout your correction. And someone that would be there to correct and/or finish things if they didn't go as planned.

I have seen many cases where patients have done an at-home treatment and are now losing teeth, have caused themselves TMJ pain and headaches, are now needing more extensive dental work, or worse. Please don't let yourself be the next victim. Don't let some publically traded company with a profit-oriented CEO steel your opportunity to Rock Your Smile!

ABOUT THE AUTHOR

Dr. Boyd O. Whitlock III received his Bachelor of Science degree in Psychology from Oklahoma State University in Stillwater, OK. He received his dental degree from University of Oklahoma College of Dentistry in Oklahoma City, OK. After dental school, Dr. Whitlock completed a one-year hospital general practice residency at Children's Hospital in Oklahoma City, OK. Following his hospital residency, Dr. Whitlock received his Masters in orthodontics from the University of Missouri-Kansas City in Kansas City, MO.

Dr. Whitlock grew up in Oklahoma. His dad was a physician (Dr. Boyd O. Whitlock Jr.) and his mom was an RN (Myrna Whitlock). Growing up in a medical family, he has been surrounded by healthcare his whole life. He wore braces four times because of abnormal jaw growth (maybe didn't wear his retainer exactly as he was suppose to, either) and had two jaw surgeries. Because of this his passion has been to continue to find ways to reduce the time in braces, make it a more enjoyable experience, improve a person's overall health, and treat everyone as a member of his Whitlock Ortho family.

An innovator and educator, Dr. Whitlock lectures to both doctors and orthodontic staff on the most advanced orthodontic treatment philosophies and techniques available. Dr. Whitlock is a faculty member and Clinical Advisory Board member at suresmile (an advanced 3D CadCam planning software and robotically bent orthodontic arch wires). He has also lectured and advised on accelerated treatment. Dr. Whitlock is a member of numerous professional organizations both locally and nationally.

Made in the USA
Monee, IL
20 November 2021

82266538R00049